Sm

25 Healthy Smoothie Recipes
for Better Health

By: Michael L. Becker

ISBN-13: 978-1481939034

PUBLISHED BY:

IMT, LLC

Please visit us at:

http://betterhealth360.com/

DISCLAIMER AND TERMS OF USE

No information contained in this book should be considered as physical, health related, financial, tax, or legal advice. Your reliance upon information and content obtained by you at or through this publication is solely at your own risk. The author assumes no liability or responsibly for damage or injury to you, other persons, or property arising from any use of any product, information, idea, or instruction contained in the content provided to you through this book.

The content and information contained in this book are for educational purposes only. These statements have not been evaluated by the Food and Drug Administration.
These statements are not intended to diagnose, treat, cure or prevent any disease. If you are pregnant, nursing, taking medication, or have a medical condition, consult your physician before using this product.

Other books in the Optimum Health Series

Juicing Delicious Juice Recipes for Optimum Health (Optimum Health Series)

Muscle Mass: The Top Reasons Your Not Growing A Complete Guide For Maximum Muscle Growth

Lose Weight 7 Pounds In 7 Days The Complete Body Transformation Guide (Optimum Health Series)

Salads 101 Simple Salad Recipes for Optimum Health (Optimum Health Series)

Michael L. Becker

Smoothies 25 Healthy Smoothie Recipes for Better Health

Introduction

I would like to thank you for purchasing one of my books. With all the misinformation out there about how to lose weight and become healthier it's no wonder that the World Health Organization (WHO) states that there are approximately 1.6 Billion people overweight in the world today. The WHO projects that that number will increase by 40% in the next 10 years. It is my goal to help as many people as possible learn how to lose weight and get in better shape by the foods we eat and in this case drink.

There's nothing like making a frozen smoothie which tastes great and provides so many macro nutrients that actually feed our bodies. You can lose weight by simply adding one of these delicious smoothies to your daily diet. The fruits and vegetables can provide your body with nutrients it craves for optimum health.

The smoothies outlined in this book are some of the top smoothies my family enjoys on a daily basis, and I hope you enjoy them too.

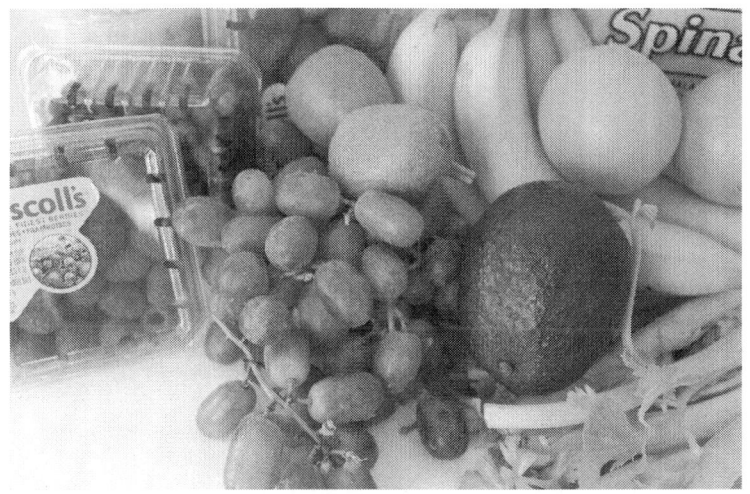

In this book, you are going to enjoy delicious whole food smoothies that taste great. It is my experience that when incorporating green vegetables in the smoothies, the vegetable flavor may be overpowering. I recommend experimenting with the amount of vegetables you add to your smoothie. If you try a recipe that contains vegetables and vegetables are too strong for your taste, simply cut back on the vegetable portion the next time you make that specific smoothie. We love knowing that the vegetables are a part of the smoothies we drink and have grown accustom to their wonderful flavor in the drinks.

Before I started juicing and making smoothies on a daily basis, I would never seem to have enough energy throughout the day. I was tired all the time and would come home from work and sit down on the couch and watch television until retiring for the evening. I just didn't have any energy to play with the kids or get involved with the families activities.

Once I bought my first juicer, I was hooked. I made a juice and was surprised at how good it actually tasted. After just one glass, I was seemed to have more energy and this started me on a daily juicing schedule. Fast forward 5 years later, I'm full of energy, more active than I was when I was 20 years old and now spend time playing with the kids, walking the dog, and spending quality time I wouldn't have had if not for feeding my body with the essential macro nutrients it needed on a daily basis.

So, now it's your turn to start enjoying the benefits of juicing with these amazingly simple but delicious smoothie recipes. Once you start feeding your body with these essential nutrients, I'm sure you will also experience more energy and rest better knowing you are feeding your body with essential nutrients necessary for optimum health.

If you enjoy this book and the wonderful delicious smoothie recipes, please consider leaving a review for this book on Amazon, so more people will see and can experience the power of juicing with smoothies.

So, once you find a smoothie recipe that sounds good to you, make sure you take out your juicer and get started today on your new healthier journey. I'm sure you'll be glad you did.

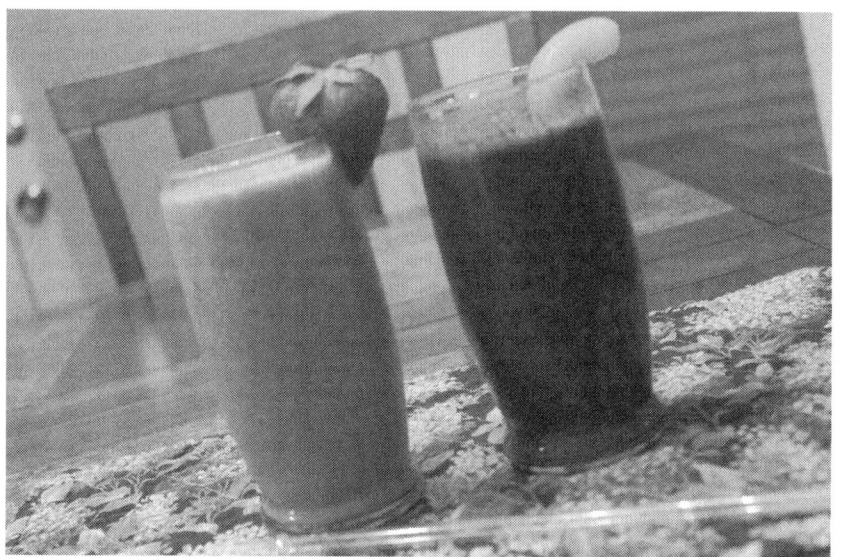

Suggested Smoothie Tools

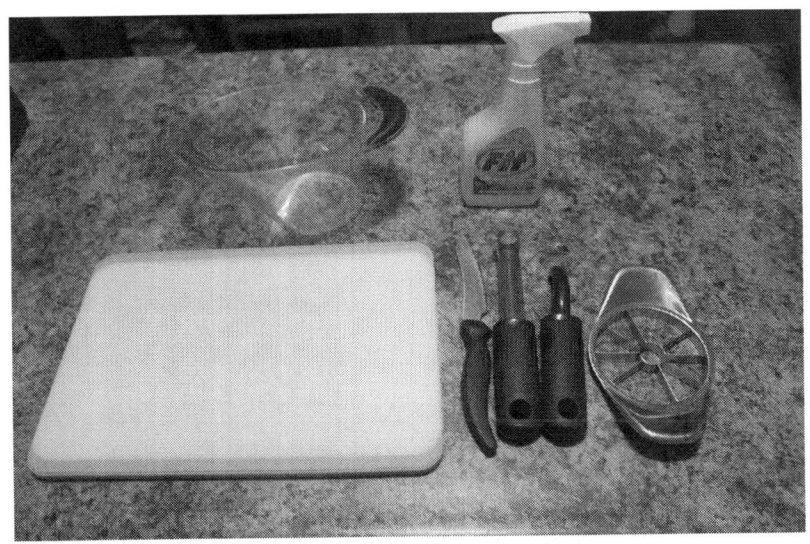

Quick Reference:

1. **Vitamix Juicer, Blendtec blender or similar type juicer and a blender**
2. **Cutting Board**
3. **Kitchen Knife**
4. **Apple Corer**
5. **Measuring Cup**
6. **Veggie & Fruit Wash – an**

example we use is Flit

Tools Explained

1. Vitamix Juicer or Blendtec Blender– I own a Vitamix juicer and all instructions and directions are written for the use of the Vitamix juicer. If you don't own one, don't worry simply juice the fruits and veggies with whatever type of juicer you do have. If your juicer separates the pulp you will simply keep the pulp and add the pulp, fresh juice and frozen fruits or ice into a blender to make the smoothie.

2. Cutting Board – the cutting board is recommended to cut fruits and veggies into smaller pieces and to core apples and any fruits or veggies that have pits, seeds, cores or anything that is hard and shouldn't be placed in your juicer. Remember to follow the directions of your particular style juicer when juicing. The cutting board will also help to protect your counter tops from any damage.

3. Kitchen Knife – I suggest making sure your favorite knife is sharp to cut fruits and veggies into smaller pieces to fit into the juicer.

4. Apple Corer – You can use a single center apple corer or an apple corer that also slices the apple into several pieces, which cuts down, on prep time.

5. Measuring Cup – The measuring cup will help measure the proper amount of fruits, veggies and other ingredient that are recommended in your specific smoothie recipe. If you are using fresh produce for your juices and no frozen fruits, you will want to add ice as this will make the smoothie thicker and cold.

6. Veggie & Fruit Wash – Any Veggie or fruit spray that is natural can be used to help wash away any pesticides, dirt and bacteria before juicing. I use a brand called "Flit" which is found at our local super market.

Next, we'll take a look at some juicing smoothie tips to help make your smoothies come out perfect.

Smoothies 25 Healthy Smoothie Recipes for Better Health

Smoothie Tips & Tricks

1.   Think about purchasing frozen fruits from your favorite discount warehouse club. Frozen fruit tends to be cheaper when purchased in bulk, can be readily available and easily stored in your freezer. By using frozen fruits you won't have to add ice to make your smoothie, the frozen fruit should be cold enough to turn your juice into a delicious smoothie without adding ice which can also cut down on pre time.

2.   Make sure to core any type of fruits that have pits, seeds, stems and peel any citrus fruits before juicing as the peel will turn the smoothie bitter.

3.   Our goal is to break all the fruits and veggies down into the smallest particles we can as fast as we can to keep the juice ice cold and smoothie texture. The longer you have the juicer or blender running, the warmer the contents of your smoothie will become which can cause the contents to become runny and have a less smoothie texture. Try and run your juicer no more than one minute when possible to get the best texture possible.

4.   These smoothie recipes taste delicious and add a lot of vitamin, minerals, phytochemicals, and fiber which the Food and Drug Administration suggests getting at least

9 servings of fresh fruits and vegetables daily. Juicing is a great way to get those fruits and vegetable, and they taste great, however, these recipes are just a base at which you can play around and create other great tasting smoothies by adding some of your other favorite great tasting ingredients.

5.   Now that you are incorporating more fruits and vegetables on a regular basis you might want to spice up your smoothies to make them more like a desert. You can easily add ice cream fruit flavored yogurts, chocolate, honey, agave, 2% or whole milk, malt powder, and any other ingredients you think would make a great tasting smoothie. These smoothies can be a

special treat you enjoy every once in a while to reward yourself for the hard work of following a better diet. We all need cheat days to stay on track with our healthy diets. I would incorporate a check meal once every 4 days as this shouldn't hurt your overall healthy diet. I suggest following a healthy diet 90% of the time and don't feel guilty for incorporating and enjoying a cheat meal here and there. Rewarding yourself for your hard work once in a while can help you stick to an overall better diet for the long haul.

6.   If the recipe you are making seems to be too large to drink in one setting or you're making a smoothie for one, simply adjust the amount of

ingredients while trying to keep the percentages of those contents close for best results.

7. To turn any smoothie recipe into a desert type smoothie, you can substitute 2 scoops of your favorite ice cream for ice cubes. You can also sweeten these smoothies with organic honey, dates, and agave.

8. You can also include a scoop or two of your favorite protein powder to increase your protein intake while creating your own masterpiece.

9. The smoothies that are listed in this book are based on mostly fruits and are very delicious and should be very enjoyable if you are just starting to incorporate juicing into your diet. There are a few smoothie recipes

toward the end of the book that also contain some vegetables. Vegetables offer an array of nutrients that may not be found in fruits and once you get accustom to fruit smoothies you might want to think about incorporating green juicing and green smoothies into your diet to get even more nutrients that only vegetables offer.

10. I suggest varying your smoothies each day as each fruit and vegetable contains different nutrients, vitamins, minerals and macro nutrients your body craves. Incorporating different types of smoothies each day, your body can receive an array of fruits and vegetable with varying amounts of different nutrients.

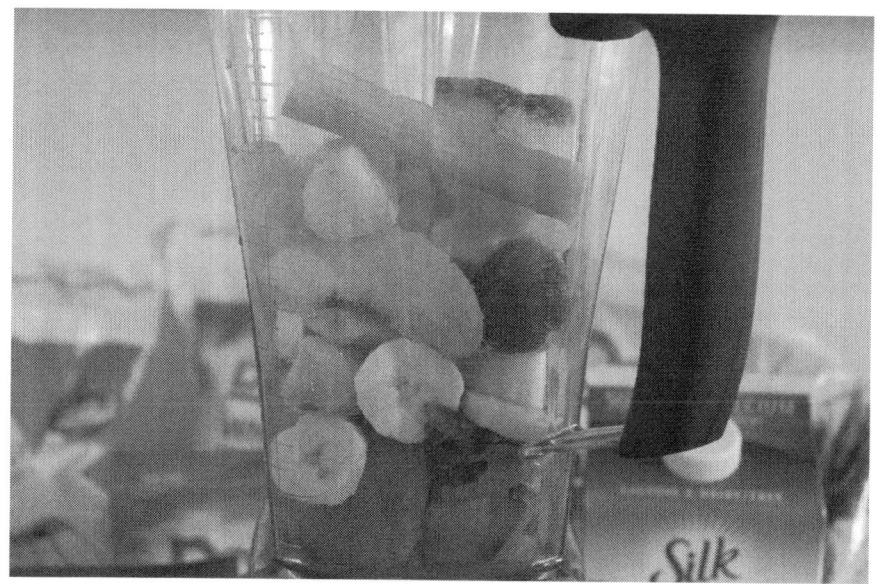

Strawberry Banana Smoothie

Preparation Time: 2 minutes

Makes: 5 cups

Ingredients:

1 pint strawberries, stemmed, washed

2 ripe bananas cut into small chunks

1 cup vanilla yogurt

3 cups milk

Directions:

1.   Place contents into juicer with the softest fruits first and then layer harder or frozen fruits towards the top.

2.   Blend on high speed for approximately 1 minute or until you

reach the desired smoothie texture, making sure all contents are blended thoroughly.

3.	Serve immediately for best results, taste and freshness.

4.	Top with your favorite fruit.

Blueberry Orange Banana Smoothie

Preparation time: 5 minutes
Makes: 2 cups

Ingredients:

½ cup frozen blueberries

1 medium orange, peeled, quartered

1 medium frozen banana, peeled

¾ cup water or I like Almond Milk for a nutty flavor and creamy texture

Directions:

1.   Place contents into juicer with the softest fruits first and then layer harder or frozen fruits towards the top.

2.   Blend on high speed for approximately 1 minute or until you reach the desired smoothie texture, making sure all contents are blended thoroughly.

3.   Serve immediately for best results, taste and freshness.

4.   Top with your favorite fruit.

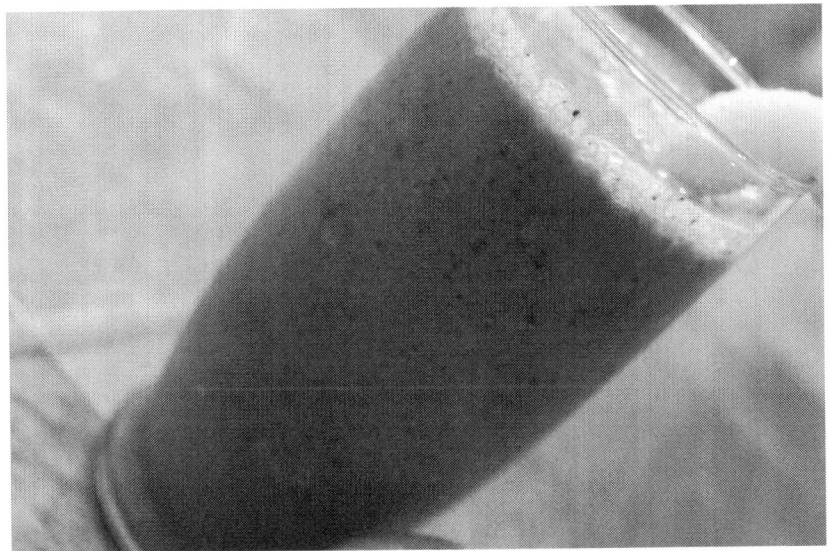

Smoothies 25 Healthy Smoothie Recipes for Better Health

Orchard Fresh Smoothie

Prep time: 5 minutes

Makes: 5 cups

Ingredients:

2 cups of your favorite colored grapes (red or green)

1 cup frozen raspberries

2 cups of frozen peaches

2 tablespoons of organic honey (for a sweeter taste)

2 cups water or Almond Milk

Directions:

1.   Place contents into juicer with the softest fruits first and then layer harder or frozen fruits towards the top.

2. Blend on high speed for approximately 1 minute or until you reach the desired smoothie texture, making sure all contents are blended thoroughly.

3. Serve immediately for best results, taste and freshness.

4. Top with your favorite fruit.

Watermelon Kiwi Smoothie

Prep time: 5 minutes

Makes: 2 3/4 cups

Ingredients:

1 ½ cups watermelon peeled, and cut into small pieces

1 kiwi, peeled, cut in half

1 date, pitted

1 cup of ice cubes

Directions:

1.   Place contents into juicer with the softest fruits first and then layer harder or frozen fruits towards the top.

2.   Blend on high speed for

approximately 1 minute or until you reach the desired smoothie texture, making sure all contents are blended thoroughly.

3.   Serve immediately for best results, taste and freshness.

4.   Top with your favorite fruit.

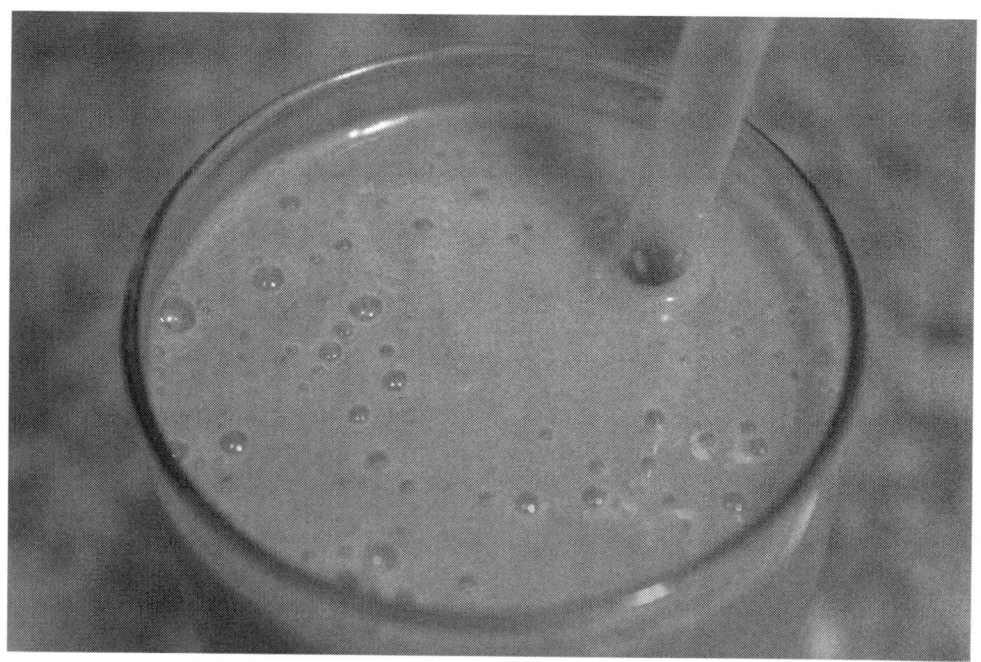

Morning Dew Smoothie

Morning Dew is an awesome smoothie to get your day started off right. Delicious morning fruits can provide a natural energy boost; you may even want to skip your morning coffee.

Prep Time: 5 minutes

Makes: 3 ¾ cups

Ingredients:

1 cup honeydew melon, cut into small pieces

½ peach, peeled, pitted

1 medium orange, peeled, quartered

½ cup fresh pineapple, cored, cut into small pieces

¼ cup water or Almond Milk (Your

preference)

1 cup ice cubes

Directions:

1.   Place contents into juicer with the softest fruits first and then layer harder or frozen fruits towards the top.

2.   Blend on high speed for approximately 1 minute or until you reach the desired smoothie texture, making sure all contents are blended thoroughly.

3.   Serve immediately for best results, taste and freshness.

4.   Top with your favorite fruit.

Sweet Mango Smoothie

Tropical fruits taste good anytime of the day. An afternoon tropical fruit smoothie may be just what you need for a great snack.

Prep time: 5 minutes

Makes: 3 cups

Ingredients:

½ mango, pitted, and peeled

½ medium sized apple, cored, and seeded

½ medium sized banana, peeled

1 medium sized orange, peeled, and quartered

1 cup ice cubes

Directions:

1.   Place contents into juicer with the softest fruits first and then layer harder or frozen fruits towards the top.

2.   Blend on high speed for approximately 1 minute or until you reach the desired smoothie texture, making sure all contents are blended thoroughly.

3.   Serve immediately for best results, taste and freshness.

4.   Top with your favorite fruit.

Summer Fruit Smoothie

Prep time: 5 minutes
Makes: 4 ½ cups

Ingredients:

½ cup cantaloupe, cut into small pieces

1 cup honeydew cut into small pieces

1 cup fresh pineapple, cut, cored, peeled

1 medium sized peach, pitted, quartered

1 cup ice cubes

1 cup water or Almond Milk

Directions:

1.   Place contents into juicer with the softest fruits first and then layer harder or frozen fruits towards the top.

2.   Blend on high speed for approximately 1 minute or until you reach the desired smoothie texture, making sure all contents are blended thoroughly.

3.   Serve immediately for best results, taste and freshness.

4.   Top with your favorite fruit.

Tropical Berry Smoothie

Prep time: 5 minutes

Makes: 3 cups

Ingredients:

½ lime, peeled, seeded

½ cup favorite colored grapes (red or green)

½ cup fresh or frozen raspberries or blackberries

½ cup pineapple, cored, peeled

1 ½ cups ice cubes

Directions:

1.   Place contents into juicer with the softest fruits first and then layer harder

or frozen fruits towards the top.

2. Blend on high speed for approximately 1 minute or until you reach the desired smoothie texture, making sure all contents are blended thoroughly.

3. Serve immediately for best results, taste and freshness.

4. Top with your favorite fruit.

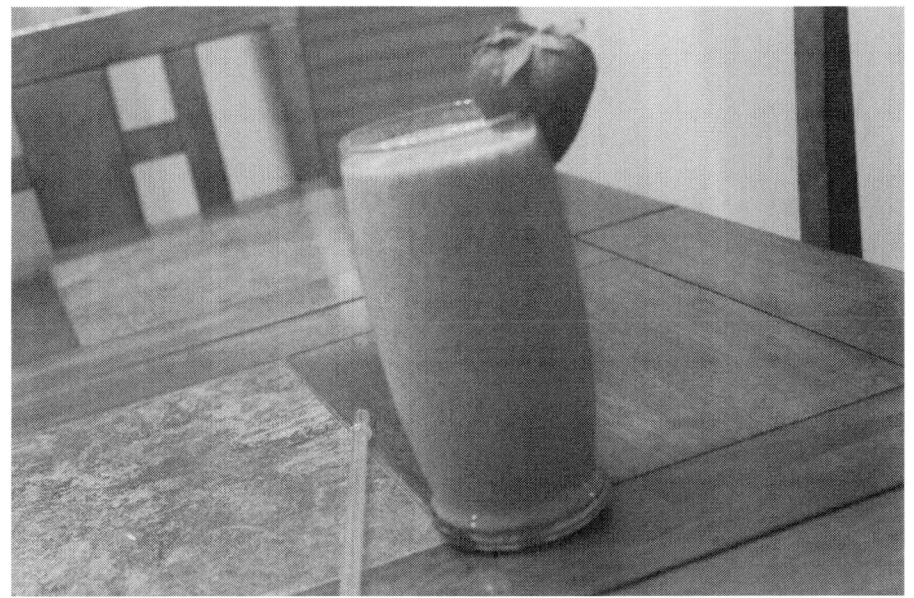

Smoothies 25 Healthy Smoothie Recipes for Better Health

Almond Berry Smoothie

You might enjoy a different type of nut with this great recipe as each nut you select can add a unique flavor to this smoothie!

Prep time: 5 minutes

Makes: 2 ½ cups

Ingredients:

½ cup fresh or frozen blackberries

½ banana, peeled

2 tablespoons almonds

1 tablespoon sunflower seeds

2 dates or 2 tablespoons of organic honey

¼ cup favorite fruit yogurt

1 cup ice cubes

½ cup of water or Almond Milk

Directions:

1.   Place contents into juicer with the softest fruits first and then layer harder or frozen fruits towards the top.

2.   Blend on high speed for approximately 1 minute or until you reach the desired smoothie texture, making sure all contents are blended thoroughly.

3.   Serve immediately for best results, taste and freshness.

4.   Top with your favorite fruit.

Smoothies 25 Healthy Smoothie Recipes for Better Health

Very Berry Smoothie

If you are looking for a lower glycemic type of smoothie, this wonderful berry smoothie will provide you with great taste while keeping the glycemic index lower.

Prep time: 5 minutes

Makes: 3 cups

Ingredients:

½ cup fresh or frozen blackberries

½ cup fresh or frozen blueberries

½ cup fresh or frozen strawberries

½ cup fresh or frozen raspberries

¼ cup favorite fruit yogurt

½ cup of water or Almond Milk

1 cup ice cubes if you decide to use

fresh fruits for smoothie texture

Directions:

1.   Place contents into juicer with the softest fruits first and then layer harder or frozen fruits towards the top.

2.   Blend on high speed for approximately 1 minute or until you reach the desired smoothie texture, making sure all contents are blended thoroughly.

3.   Serve immediately for best results, taste and freshness.

4.   Top with your favorite fruit.

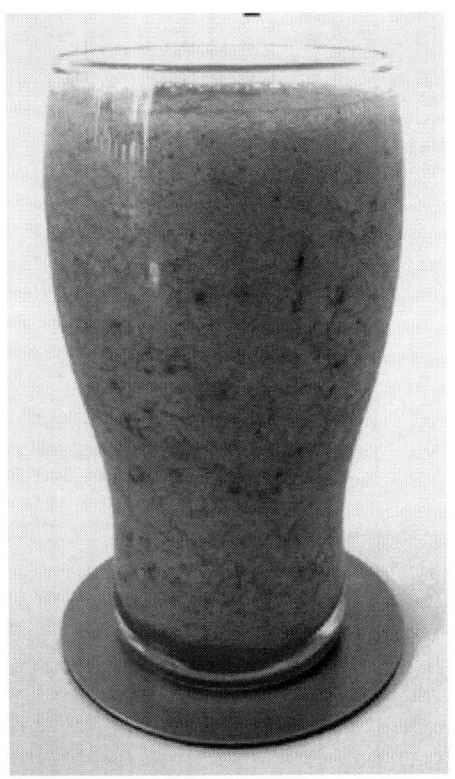

Berry Blast Smoothie

You may enjoy adding an banana, apple, or pineapple to this great drink. A medium ripe banana, 1 medium apple or 1 cup of pineapple can naturally sweeten this delicious smoothie. You might even try adding some organic honey.

Prep time: 5 minutes

Makes: 3 cups

Ingredients:

1/3 cup fresh or frozen cranberries

½ cup fresh or frozen blueberries

1cup fresh or frozen strawberries

1 medium banana, peeled

1 cup pineapple, cut into small pieces, cored

½ cup ice cubes

Directions:

1.   Place contents into juicer with the softest fruits first and then layer harder or frozen fruits towards the top.

2.   Blend on high speed for approximately 1 minute or until you reach the desired smoothie texture, making sure all contents are blended thoroughly.

3.   Serve immediately for best results, taste and freshness.

4.   Top with your favorite fruit.

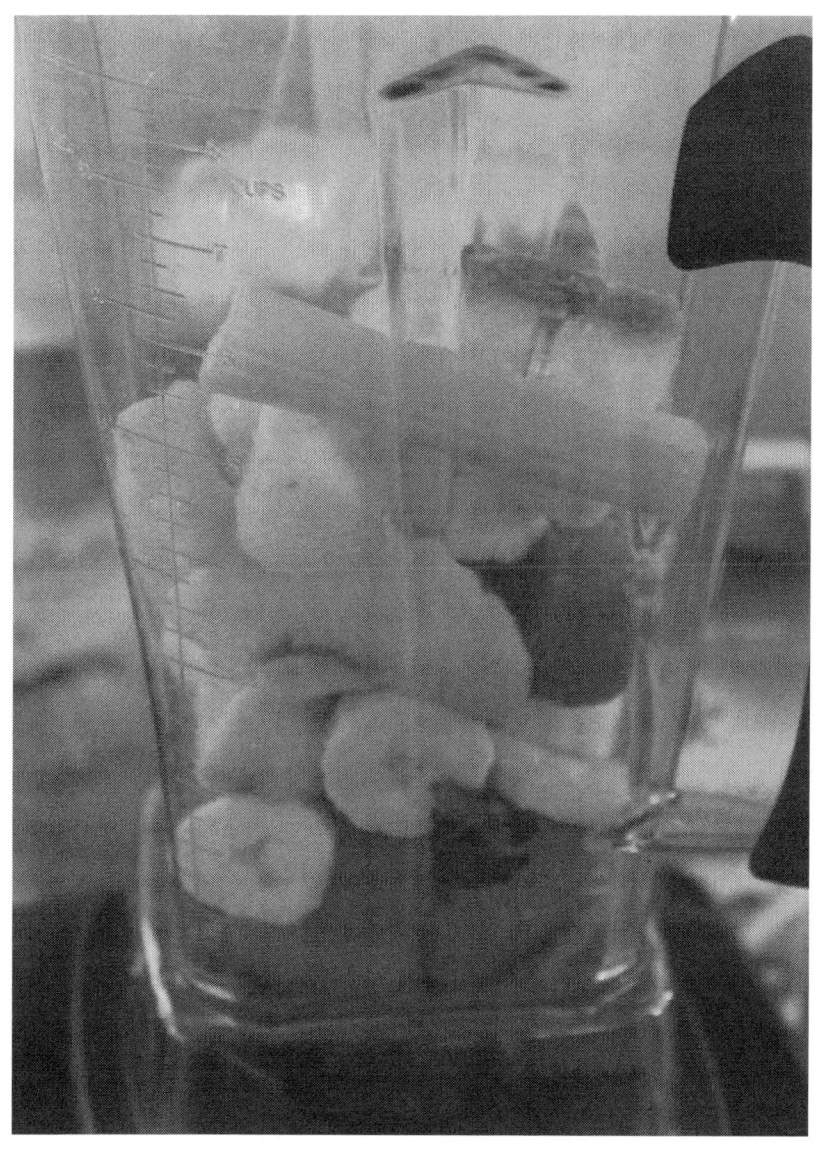

Smoothies 25 Healthy Smoothie Recipes for Better Health

Mango Peach Delight Smoothie

Prep time: 5 minutes

Makes: 2 cups

Ingredients:

1 medium sized peach, peeled, pitted

½ mango, peeled, pitted

1 tablespoon organic honey or 2 dates

½ cup water or Almond Milk

1 cup ice cubes

Directions:

1.   Place contents into juicer with the softest fruits first and then layer harder or frozen fruits towards the top.

2.   Blend on high speed for approximately 1 minute or until you reach the desired smoothie texture, making sure all contents are blended thoroughly.

3.   Serve immediately for best results, taste and freshness.

4.   Top with your favorite fruit.

Blueberry Peach Smoothie

Prep time: 5 minutes

Makes: 2 ½ cups

Ingredients:

1 cup blueberries, fresh or frozen

1 medium peach, pitted, quartered

½ cup favorite color grapes (red or green)

1 cup ice cubes

Directions:

1. Place contents into juicer with the softest fruits first and then layer harder or frozen fruits towards the top.

2.   Blend on high speed for approximately 1 minute or until you reach the desired smoothie texture, making sure all contents are blended thoroughly.

3.   Serve immediately for best results, taste and freshness.

4.   Top with your favorite fruit.

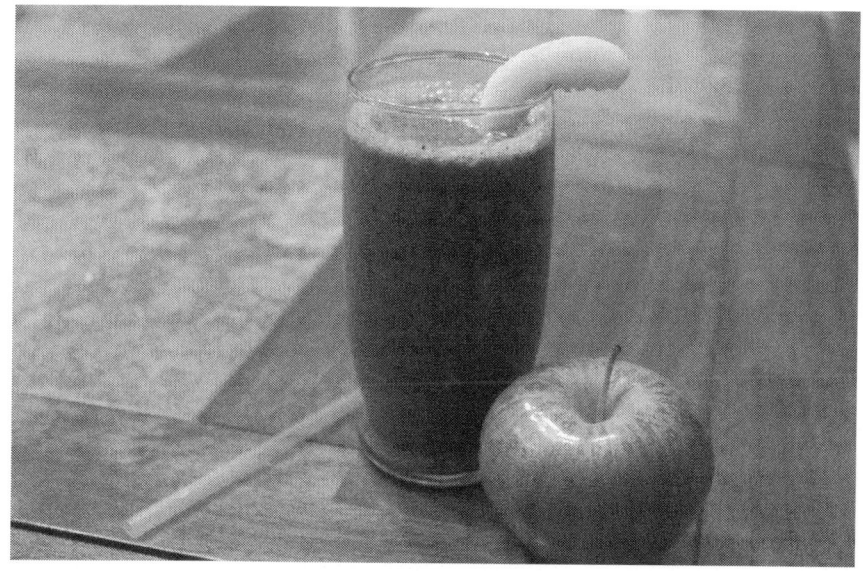

Minty Cherry Lime Smoothie

This smoothie will surely bring your taste buds to life. You will get a minty, tart flavor than can be toned down slightly by adding some Almond Milk.

Prep time: 5 minutes

Makes: 2 ½ cups

Ingredients:

¼ medium lime, peeled, seeded

1 cup fresh or frozen cherries

3 medium mint leaves

1 cup ice cubes

¾ cup Almond Milk

Directions:

1.   Place contents into juicer with the softest fruits first and then layer harder or frozen fruits towards the top.

2.   Blend on high speed for approximately 1 minute or until you reach the desired smoothie texture, making sure all contents are blended thoroughly.

3.   Serve immediately for best results, taste and freshness.

4.   Top with your favorite fruit.

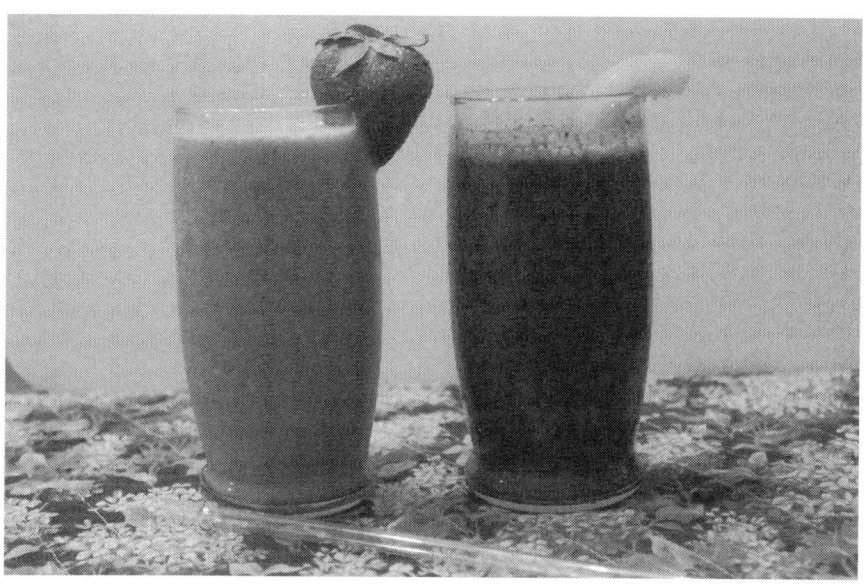

Smoothies 25 Healthy Smoothie Recipes for Better Health

Strawberry Mango Smoothie

Prep time: 5 minutes

Makes: 3 cups

Ingredients:

1 cup fresh or frozen Strawberries

1 cup fresh or frozen Mangoes

1 cup vanilla yogurt

1/3 cup organic honey

3 cups low-fat milk

1 cup crushed ice

Directions:

1.   Place contents into juicer with the softest fruits first and then layer harder

or frozen fruits towards the top.

2.   Blend on high speed for approximately 1 minute or until you reach the desired smoothie texture, making sure all contents are blended thoroughly.

3.   Serve immediately for best results, taste and freshness.

4.   Top with your favorite fruit.

Raspberry Peach Smoothie

Prep time: 5 minutes

Makes: 3 cups

Ingredients:

1/2 cup fresh or frozen raspberries

1 cup fresh or frozen peach slices

1 medium apple, cored

1/2 cup vanilla yogurt

1 cup ice cubes

Directions:

1.   Place contents into juicer with the softest fruits first and then layer harder or frozen fruits towards the top.

2.   Blend on high speed for approximately 1 minute or until you reach the desired smoothie texture, making sure all contents are blended thoroughly.

3.   Serve immediately for best results, taste and freshness.

4.   Top with your favorite fruit.

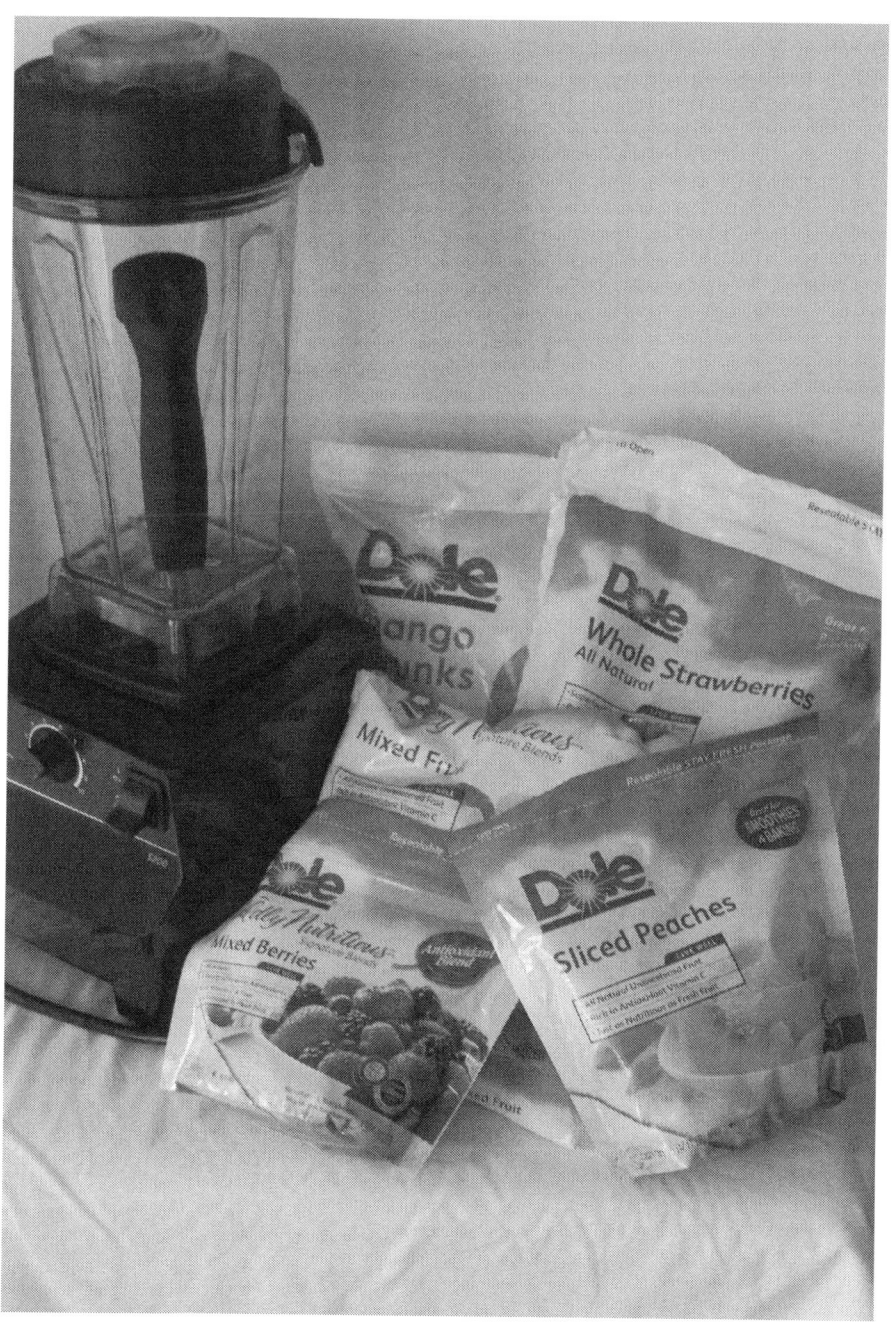

Smoothies 25 Healthy Smoothie Recipes for Better Health

Kiwi Lime Surprise Smoothie

If you love Key Lime pie, I'm sure you will love a Kiwi, Lime Surprise Smoothie. What a healthy, natural alternative this delicious smoothie will be.

Prep time: 5 minutes

Makes: 2 cups

Ingredients:

2 Kiwis, peeled, quartered

1 large pear, quartered

1 tablespoon key lime juice

2 tablespoons organic honey or 2 dates

¼ cup water or Almond Milk

1 cup ice cubes

Directions:

1.   Place contents into juicer with the softest fruits first and then layer harder or frozen fruits towards the top.

2.   Blend on high speed for approximately 1 minute or until you reach the desired smoothie texture, making sure all contents are blended thoroughly.

3.   Serve immediately for best results, taste and freshness.

4.   Top with your favorite fruit.

Chocolate Banana Smoothie

Prep time: 5 minutes

Makes: 3 cups

Ingredients:

1 large banana fresh or frozen, peeled, cut into small pieces

1 cup vanilla yogurt

2 tablespoons favorite chocolate syrup (There are some great fat-free choices to choose from).

¾ cup Almond Milk or skim milk

1 cup ice cubes

Directions:

1.   Place contents into juicer with the softest fruits first and then layer harder or frozen fruits towards the top.

2.   Blend on high speed for approximately 1 minute or until you reach the desired smoothie texture, making sure all contents are blended thoroughly.

3.   Serve immediately for best results, taste and freshness.

4.   Top with your favorite fruit.

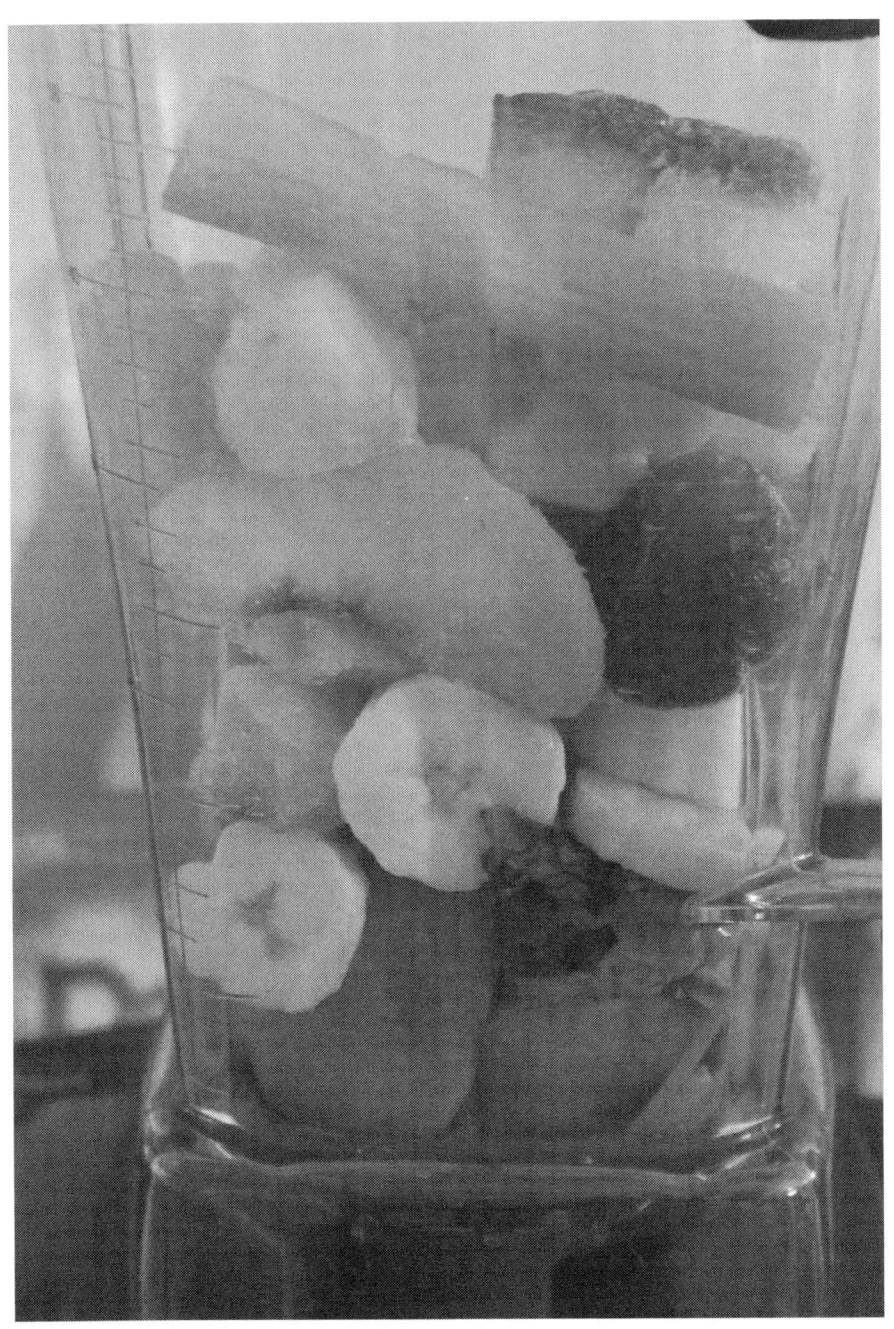

Smoothies 25 Healthy Smoothie Recipes for Better Health

Healthy Green Smoothie

Try incorporating small amounts of greens into your smoothies to better alkalize your body. If you're not used to drinking green drinks, it is better to start with small amounts and increase the green vegetables as you become accustomed to their flavors.

Prep time: 5 minutes
Makes: 3 cups

Ingredients:

½ cup pineapple, cored, cut into small pieces

¼ pear, cored, stemmed

1 ½ cups green grapes, stemmed

1 broccoli top

½ cup spinach, washed

½ small avocado, peeled, pitted

½ cup water or Almond Milk

1 cup ice cubes

Directions:

1.   Place contents into juicer with the softest fruits first and then layer harder or frozen fruits towards the top.

2.   Blend on high speed for approximately 1 minute or until you reach the desired smoothie texture, making sure all contents are blended thoroughly.

3.   Serve immediately for best results, taste and freshness.

4.   Top with your favorite fruit.

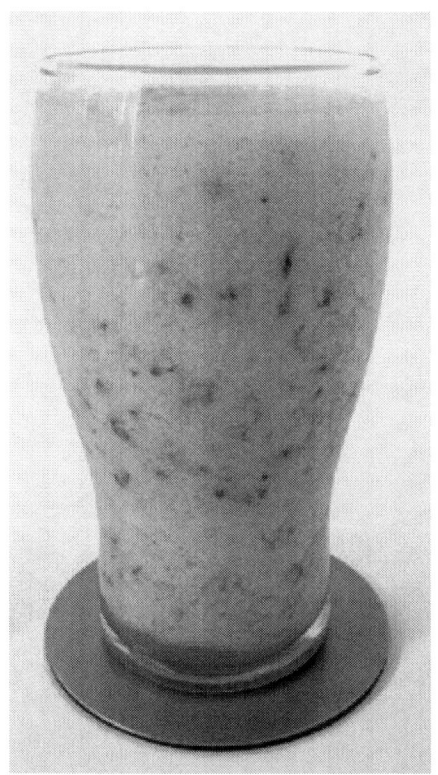

Sunrise Energy Smoothie

Prep time: 5 minutes

Makes: 3 cups

Ingredients:

½ medium apple, cored, quartered

¼ small lemon, peeled, seeded

½ kiwi, peeled, quartered

1 cup green grapes, stemmed

¼ cup cucumber, peeled, cut into small pieces

¾ cup organic broccoli tops, cut into small pieces

½ cup water

1 cup ice cubes

Directions:

1. Place contents into juicer with the softest fruits first and then layer harder or frozen fruits towards the top.

2. Blend on high speed for approximately 1 minute or until you reach the desired smoothie texture, making sure all contents are blended thoroughly.

3. Serve immediately for best results, taste and freshness.

4. Top with your favorite fruit.

Tropical Green Smoothie

Prep time: 5 minutes

Makes: 5 cups

Ingredients:

1 cup fresh or frozen strawberries

2 medium fresh or frozen bananas, peeled

2 cups organic fresh spinach, washed

1 cup Almond Milk or skim milk

1 cup ice cubes

Directions:

1. Place contents into juicer with the softest fruits first and then layer harder or frozen fruits towards the top.

2. Blend on high speed for

approximately 1 minute or until you reach the desired smoothie texture, making sure all contents are blended thoroughly.

3.   Serve immediately for best results, taste and freshness.

4.   Top with your favorite fruit.

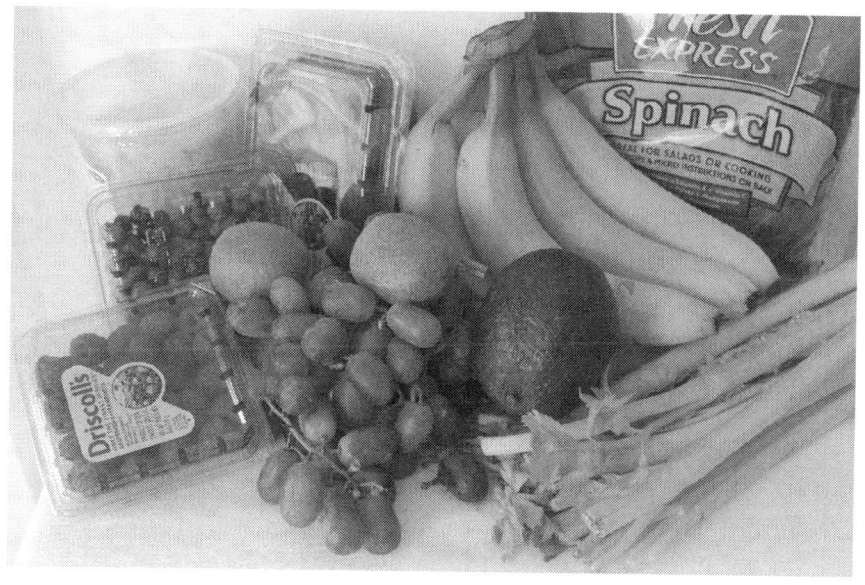

Smoothies 25 Healthy Smoothie Recipes for Better Health

Tangy Tropical Smoothie

Prep time: 5 minutes

Makes: 4 cups

Ingredients:

2 medium apples, cored, cut into small pieces

1 medium fresh or frozen banana, peeled

½ lime, peeled

1 cup organic spinach, washed

½ cup Almond Milk or water

1 cup ice cubes

Directions:

1.   Place contents into juicer with the softest fruits first and then layer harder

or frozen fruits towards the top.

2.   Blend on high speed for approximately 1 minute or until you reach the desired smoothie texture, making sure all contents are blended thoroughly.

3.   Serve immediately for best results, taste and freshness.

4.   Top with your favorite fruit.

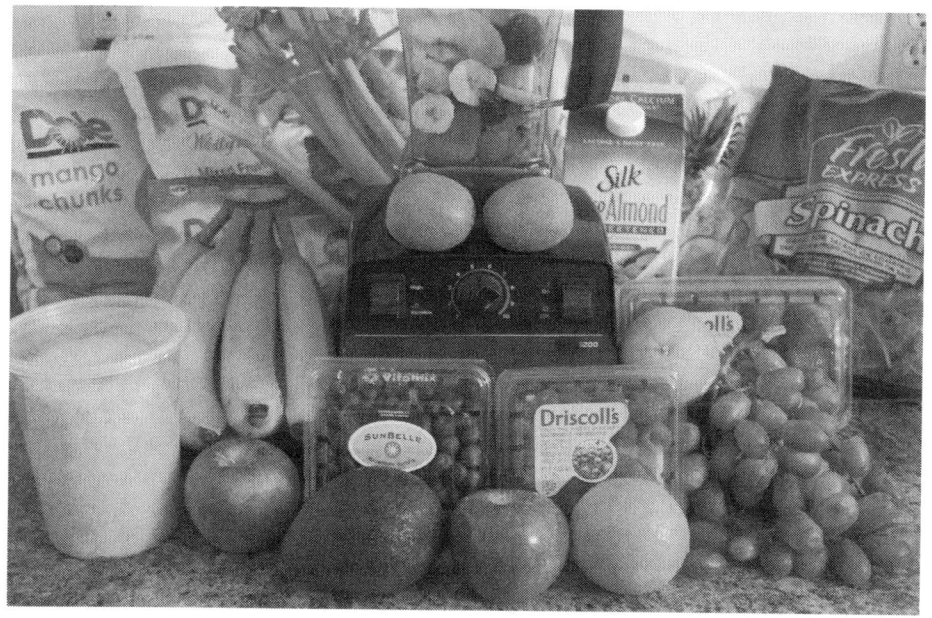

Smoothies 25 Healthy Smoothie Recipes for Better Health

Peanut Butter Banana Smoothie

The only thing missing in this delicious smoothie is the jelly. Well, I simply love the ingredients in this smoothie. If you prefer, you might enjoy substituting smooth peanut butter for crunchy peanut butter.

Prep time: 5 minutes

Makes: 4 cups

Ingredients:

2 tablespoons favorite crunchy peanut butter

2 fresh or frozen ripe bananas, peeled, cut into small pieces

1 1/2 cups Almond Milk or skim milk

1/4 cup vanilla yogurt

1 tablespoon of organic honey

1 tablespoon wheat germ

1 cup ice cubes

Directions:

1. Place contents into juicer with the softest fruits first and then layer harder or frozen fruits towards the top.

2. Blend on high speed for approximately 1 minute or until you reach the desired smoothie texture, making sure all contents are blended thoroughly.

3. Serve immediately for best results, taste and freshness.

4. Once served, add honey to taste.

5. Substitute 2 scoops of vanilla ice cream for the 1 cup of ice cubes for a thicker, creamier smoothie.

6. Add healthy cinnamon for slightly different taste.

7. Top with a couple slices of banana

and/or a tablespoon of peanut butter.

Berry Grape Smoothie

Prep time: 5 minutes

Makes: 5 cups

Ingredients:

1 cup fresh or frozen strawberries

1 cup fresh or frozen blueberries

1 cup red grapes, stemmed

1 cup green grapes, stemmed

1 cup ice cubes

½ cup Almond Milk or skim milk

Directions:

1.   Place contents into juicer with the softest fruits first and then layer harder or frozen fruits towards the top.

2.   Blend on high speed for approximately 1 minute or until you reach the desired smoothie texture, making sure all contents are blended thoroughly.

3.   Serve immediately for best results, taste and freshness.

4.   Can substitute scoops of ice cream for 1 cup of ice cubes for creamier smoothie.

5.   Top with your favorite fruit.

Banana Passion Smoothie

Prep time: 5 minutes

Makes: 4 cups

Ingredients:

2 large fresh or frozen bananas, peeled, cut into small pieces

1 passion fruit, pulp removed, cut into small pieces to garnish

3/4 cup Almond Milk or skim milk

2 scoops vanilla ice-cream

1 cup vanilla yogurt

2 tablespoons vanilla Italian flavored syrup

Directions:

1.   Place contents into juicer with the softest fruits first and then layer harder or frozen fruits towards the top.

2.   Blend on high speed for approximately 1 minute or until you reach the desired smoothie texture, making sure all contents are blended thoroughly.

3.   Serve immediately for best results, taste and freshness.

4.   Top with your favorite fruit.

Final Words

I hope you enjoyed this book and have started incorporating smoothies into your daily diet like my family, and I have. Incorporating these delicious smoothies is a great way to get more vitamins, nutrients, phytochemicals, and macro nutrients in your diet in a quick and easy manner, and besides they taste delicious.

Remember these recipes are a base for you to play around with and have fun creating your own nutritious variations of these delicious recipes.

Throw out all the rules and go crazy because there are no mistakes with smoothies. If one recipes doesn't quite taste right, simply add more of your favorite fruits to taste or a little of your favorite sweeteners to make your smoothie taste even better.

If you enjoyed reading this book, and believe it will help improve your overall health, can I encourage you to leave a review? Simply locate this book in Amazon. Scroll down the book page and click on "Write a customer review."

I would like to thank you for reviewing this book in advance, and I wish you all the best in your quest for better health.

Other Recommended Books for Optimum Health

Salads 101 Simple Salad Recipes for Optimum Health (Optimum Health Series)

Juicing Delicious Juice Recipes for Optimum Health (Optimum Health Series)

Muscle Mass: The Top Reasons Your Not Growing A Complete Guide For Maximum Muscle Growth

Lose Weight 7 Pounds In 7 Days The Complete Body Transformation Guide (Optimum Health Series)

I wish you all the best in your journey of achieving the body and health you deserve.

I have more health information on my website http://betterhealth360.com/ and would love for you to drop by and say hi sometime. Please drop by anytime and check out the latest information on how to improve your health.

If there is anything you'd like to see, be sure to leave a message while you're there.

Made in the USA
Lexington, KY
11 October 2013